T0144412

BASIC HEALTH
PUBLICATIONS
USER'S GUIDE

TO
BRAIN-
BOOSTING
SUPPLEMENTS

Learn About the Vitamins
and Other Nutrients That
Can Boost Your Memory
and End Mental
Fuzziness.

JAMES J. GORMLEY AND
SHARI LIEBERMAN, PH.D., C.N.S., F.A.C.N.
JACK CHALLEM Series Editor

The information contained in this book is based upon the research and personal and professional experiences of the author. It is not intended as a substitute for consulting with your physician or other healthcare provider. Any attempt to diagnose and treat an illness should be done under the direction of a healthcare professional.

The publisher does not advocate the use of any particular healthcare protocol but believes the information in this book should be available to the public. The publisher and author are not responsible for any adverse effects or consequences resulting from the use of the suggestions, preparations, or procedures discussed in this book. Should the reader have any questions concerning the appropriateness of any procedures or preparations mentioned, the author and the publisher strongly suggest consulting a professional healthcare advisor.

Series Editor: Jack Challem
Editor: Laura Jorstad
Typesetter: Gary A. Rosenberg
Series Cover Designer: Mike Stromberg

Basic Health Publications User's Guides are published by Basic Health Publications, Inc.
www.basichealthpub.com

ISBN: 978-1-59120-090-1 (Pbk.)
ISBN: 978-1-68162-841-7 (Hardcover)

CONTENTS

INTRODUCTION

Memory. Concentration. Mental alertness. It's probably a safe bet that these markers of brain health are really "top of mind" with you. Let's take a look at what cognition and memory are and why so many of us today are deeply concerned about the functioning of that unattractive yet all-important organ that sits between our ears.

We can't talk about memory without talking about cognition. So what is cognition? *Stedman's Medical Dictionary* describes *cognition* as "a generic term embracing the quality of knowing, which includes perceiving, recognizing, conceiving, judging, sensing, reasoning and imagining." More than that, in 1999 the U.S. Surgeon General wrote that *cognition* takes in "intelligence, language, learning and memory." That's a whole lot of territory for workings that are so dependent on proper nutrition.

Some experts believe our brains are overtaxed today. Very few would disagree that we have moved beyond the Information Age into what we might now call the "Age of Information Overload." It is believed that our cognitive processing, and maybe even our memory storage capacity itself, can become overburdened as we age. In fact, in a 2000 issue of *Medical Hypotheses*, British researcher Robin Clarke suggests that today's information saturation overtaxes our longer-term memory storage, which in turn helps bring on age-associated senile dementia and Alzheimer's disease.

There's little doubt that all of us are, to one extent or another, bombarded by work and personal e-mail, Internet spam and junk mail, faxes, magazines, twenty-four-hour news, wireless calls, digital pagers, telemarketers, and even the arcane logistics of play-date scheduling for the kids after school.

While this book won't necessarily help you simplify your life, it will help you learn about brain-boosting supplements that have a rock-solid foundation in the science of nutrition.

Nutrition is indeed the master key to brain function. Inadequate nutrition burdens our minds even further, since it is nutrition itself that can help us mentally cope with all the demands placed on us by the Information Overload society. The Surgeon General notes, "Accumulating evidence from human and animal research finds that lifestyle [including diet] modifies genetic risk in influencing the outcomes of aging."

As we age, then, nutrition is critical. In fact, the brain is completely dependent on glucose taken in a more complex form from the food we eat, says Dr. Mary McGrane in a chapter she wrote in the landmark textbook *Biochemical and Physiological Aspects of Human Nutrition* (2000).

Cognition is sensitive to a wide variety of nutritional factors. As we will outline in this book, modern nutritional science is uncovering that we can improve our mental powers effectively, and even powerfully, through a wide array of nutrients and supplements, including antioxidants, herbs, fats, and other targeted dietary supplements.

Why were we inspired to write a book about memory-boosting supplements? Both of us have been passionately communicating to people about nutritional approaches to optimal (absolutely best possible) health for years. One of us, James Gormley (JG), is an award-winning health and nutrition journalist who was editor in chief of *Better Nutrition* magazine from 1995 through 2002 and author of a 1999 book about a brain-boosting nutrient, *DHA, A Good Fat.* Shari Lieberman, Ph.D., C.N.S., F.A.C.N. (SL), is a renowned nutritionist in private practice and author of the runaway best-selling health books *The Real Vitamin & Mineral Book* (1997/2003) and *Dare to Lose: 4 Simple Steps to a Better Body* (2003). Neither of us has ever accepted the conventional dogma of the "Medical Establishment" that tells us that the body and mind are on an inexorably accelerating decline after age thirty. We don't buy that.

One of the major complaints I (SL) see in my patients after age forty is memory problems, and when they start to notice changes, they panic— this memory mania has been the subject of many of the most common letters I (JG) have received from readers.

But there's no reason to panic! The good news is that science has proven that a well-designed nutritional supplementation regimen, along with a healthy diet and sensible exercise program, significantly boosts brain performance and memory.

Our book offers a customizable approach to improving all of the areas that make up cognition, including memory. We recognize that "one size does not fit all," so we outline the supplements out there that can be tried, one by one, along with an improved diet and exercise program. Chapters 2 through 4 will take you through research on how supplements, especially antioxidants, can help nourish your mind (as well as your body) and serve as an "anti-rust" treatment for brain and body.

Chapters 5 and 6 will focus on the powerful science behind herbs and specialized supplements, and how these targeted products can provide remarkable improvement in your cognitive functions and protection against potential mental decline.

And finally, Chapters 7 through 9 will tie all the research together into a compelling whole, to wit: a holistic, diet-, exercise-, and supplement-focused program based on both the promise of cutting-edge science and the wisdom of established knowledge. You'll start off seeing why fortifying your antioxidant defense arsenal will help hold off the body's equivalent to what metal does when left outside in the rain—*rust*. Our responsible approach to memory boosting will offer real hope, not hokum, for all of you reading this and your loved ones—for anyone who feels that he or she may be experiencing mild to moderate mental fogginess, dulled concentration, and reduced memory effectiveness.

There are no magic bullets here, nor hard-to-follow diets—the *User's Guide to Brain-Boosting Supplements* just offers you what we hope is the best, most concise, practical guide to memory-boosting supplements that you are likely to find—*anywhere*.

CHAPTER 1

WHAT BRAIN-BOOSTING SUPPLEMENTS CAN HELP US ACHIEVE

*W*here did I leave my keys? Who am I sup- posed to call again? What did I mean by that scribbled note, anyway?

Everybody experiences these incidents of for- getfulness. As you age, these kinds of memory lapses can become routine, and are casually attributed to "advancing years" by many baby boomers, according to Dr. Heidi White, assistant professor of geriatric medicine at Duke University Medical Center.

Age isn't the only factor in memory loss, how- ever, says White. She notes that among possible causes for cognitive decline are medications (such as sedatives, which can dull the mind), depression (which affects concentration), and hearing or vision impairment.

In addition to that, a study out of Duke University with 165 healthy men and women, ages fifty-five through eighty-five, suggests that the ApoE4 gene may be tied to more rapid age- related brain changes (aging), even in those who have not yet been diagnosed with any brain disease.

ApoE4 Gene
Having two copies of this gene increases the chances for devel- oping pre-age-seventy Alzheimer's disease symptoms by 800 percent.

Duke University's Murali Doraiswamy says, "By understanding how this particular gene exerts its effects on the brain we might be able to come up with simple ways, such as dietary changes . . .

to try to maintain our brains in a healthier state a lot longer."

Baby Boomers and the Battle for the Mind

Keeping the brain healthy much longer is a goal of many of you, especially people who, as of this writing, are forty to fifty-eight years old—otherwise called baby boomers. If you consider that a baby boomer turns fifty every nine seconds, that means that by the year 2024 there will be 115 million people over age fifty in the United States.

Today more than 77 million people, almost 30 percent of the total United States population, were not only born between 1946 and 1964 but are, say demographers and researchers, greatly concerned about loss of memory and the aging of the mind.

According to New Jersey–based researcher Dr. Vladimir Badmaev, good memory is an "asset in the competitive struggle within the context of our social and professional lives." Poor memory, on the other hand, is associated with aging and the overall decline of mental faculties and physical health. A mind robbed of its memory, adds Badmaev, results in a dramatic and total loss of a person's identity.

Failing memory is different from the forgetfulness of a busy person or the stereotypical absent-minded professor. True failing memory is often accompanied by a person's declining sense of well-being, and is often described by symptoms such as a lack of mental clarity (brain fog), altered mood (as in depression), decreased mental abilities, worsening sleep patterns, and declining overall energy.

The Dragons of Memory

Where the brain's memory centers are located is

not a Darwinian accident. Your core memory "processors" are situated in the parts of the human brain that developed the earliest in our evolutionary flight past, in Carl Sagan's term, the Dragons of Eden. These memory matrices formed there to ensure human survival, which is the case with other vital command-and-control functions that are next-door neighbors, such as our sensory (touch, smell, hearing, sight) control centers.

Researchers have divided memory into declarative and nondeclarative. *Declarative memory* is memory as most of us understand it: remembering someone (a face) or a thing (where we put our car keys) in a conscious way. *Nondeclarative memory,* on the other hand, cannot be tapped into by direct recollection, or remembering, and is responsible for your mind's memory of very basic survival skills, coordinated movement, fight-or-flight reactions, and the long-ingrained rote memorization associated with skills and basic tasks. In the case of Alzheimer's disease, the decline of declarative memory is eventually, in late stages, followed by an inability to take care of oneself that is associated with the loss of non-declarative memory.

Of Wear and Tear and Brains Aging Gracefully

The memory-improving supplements and strategies that you will be reading about in this book are geared to the declarative-type memory that is typically associated with the wear and tear of aging and transient and chronic factors affecting it, such as nutrition and arteriosclerosis. In fact, the loss of mental adaptability, also called neuronal plasticity, may truly be due to wear and tear on physical components of the nervous system.

Although there are cumulative challenges to memory over time, introduced by the very process of aging, it's nice to know that your brain's aging isn't all bad. In 2001, at a medical conference in Berlin, researchers presented evidence that "with increasing age, people actually make better use of different regions of their brains for information processing." Positron emission tomography (PET) and other techniques show that cognitive processes become more complex as you get older. So the brain can age well as long as nutrition is the very best it can be, considering the demands placed on it by the body and the nutrient requirements it places on us.

The Brain—A High-Maintenance Organ

Since the brain (along with the liver, kidneys, and heart) runs at a metabolic rate that is fifteen to forty times faster than resting muscle tissue and fifty to one hundred times faster than fat tissue, it's not surprising that the brain's blood-flow requirements, and nutrient delivery needs, are very great.

In fact, according to Malcolm Watford and Alan G. Goodridge in *Biochemical and Physiological Aspects of Human Nutrition,* "The brain must receive a constant supply of fuel."

In addition to nutritional energy, White suggests that regular exercise for both the body and mind helps optimize cognitive function. "I think common sense would tell us," she says, "that it's important to pursue physical exercise and that it's also important to stay active cognitively."

Too, few doubt the essentiality of physical exercise to a cognition-boosting program, fending off as it does the so-called hardening of the arteries (arteriosclerosis) often associated with aging. Mental exercise is important, too.

One such approach to doing "aerobics" for the muscle between the ears is called Neurobics. According to Dr. Lawrence Katz, this is based on scientific evidence revealing that as you get older, the brain has a tremendous capacity to reorganize and "rewire" itself, and can literally forge new neural connections in its different sensory structures—if you regularly stimulate your senses by new smells, new mental challenges, and new ways of doing things (routines) that you would otherwise just do robotically every day.

Taken together, then, our brain-boosting program combines diet, supplementation, and exercise into a holistic approach to improve the quality of your mind and, hence, the quality of your life.

Today's collective nightmare of what the new millennium's extended life span could mean, worst case, is filled with real-life and celluloid images of our elders as mental vegetables kept alive by drugs, surgery, and the sterile, cocoon-like protections afforded by nursing homes and hospitals.

As baby boomers, many of us want to exorcise those dark visions. We reject the specter of ourselves with glazed eyes and on life support, and instead envision a bright future for ourselves, and those we love, defined by health—yes, *optimal* health—vigor, energy, and quality of mind.

Quality of Mind Equals Quality of Life

Since quality of mind is then, truly, at the elemental core of quality of life, ways in which you can improve your mental abilities and functions, and fend off the memory and general cognitive declines associated with aging, should be more than welcome—especially when these ways, out-

lined in the following chapters, are holistic, nutri-
ent-based, and without the profound unwanted
side effects often associated with synthetic phar-
maceutical drugs.

CHAPTER 2

ANTIOXIDANT VITAMINS

You are constantly exposed to a wide range of compounds called xenobiotics, basically the body's version of evil aliens from outer space: toxic, destructive, and cancer-causing chemicals.

Many of these chemicals are in the human diet. They can react with large cellular molecules (macromolecules), such as proteins and DNA, or directly with cell structures to cause damage. On top of this, some naturally nonreactive chemicals can be biologically morphed into reactive molecules inside cells.

Free Radicals—And We Don't Mean the Kind That Wear Tie-Dyed Shirts

Free radicals (reactive oxygen species) are produced as a normal byproduct of the body's workings. Unfortunately, environmental factors, such as cigarette smoke, polluted air, chlorinated hydrocarbons (which used to be found in all aerosol sprays), heavy metals, sunlight, and x-rays cause excess free radicals to be formed in the body.

Antioxidants
Vitamins, minerals, enzymes, or other compounds that help us fight off the formation of free radicals and the damage caused by them.

The two main defense systems your body uses to fight these free radicals are detoxification enzymes and antioxidant systems.

If Oxidation Equals Rust . . .

You know the reddish coating on metal caused by oxidation as "rust." Oxidation is important in nutrition, too, because oxidation of fats affects how food tastes and because the oxidative products that result from what is called lipid (fat) peroxidation are toxic—lipid peroxidation being the nasty process that begins when a harmless fatty acid becomes involved with oxygen, gives rise to a bad peroxyl free radical, and can wind up spiraling out of control in a cascade of new free radical "rusting" reactions.

Is All Oxidation Bad?

No. First, in most oxidative reactions it's even Steven: A balanced number of electrons are transferred, so no free radicals are formed. In addition to that, some metabolic activities actually require that free-radical-producing, reactive species be formed as part of a process to produce or eliminate certain compounds.

For example, hydrogen peroxide (H_2O_2) is by and large a bad-boy reactive oxygen species, but hydrogen peroxide is actually required for us to make the thyroid hormone thyroxine, and also needed to produce bacterium-killing hypochlorous acid in neutrophils. In these cases, the generation of free radicals is carefully controlled and compartmentalized, in order to protect other cells and tissues; our cells are further protected, in this process, by detoxification enzymes.

Our cells' energy-producing factories, mitochondria, factor in, too. Mitochondria happen to use most of the body's oxygen in a process that produces water. This is normally fine. However, a small percentage of the oxygen is transformed into reactive oxygen free radicals as a byproduct of this activity.

Toxic and synthetic chemicals, infectious germs (bad bacteria and viruses), and genetic defects that interfere with normal functioning dramatically increase the amount of oxygen that is converted into free radicals. Aging, alcohol use, drugs, and environmental toxins accelerate this process even further.

Free radicals can damage any cells and tissue, not just fat cells, and can cause changes (and mutations) in our DNA, too. These changes can add up to deterioration in the body that's associated with the signs of aging and with chronic diseases such as hardening of the arteries, arthritis, heart and kidney ailments, and even cancer. These nasty free radicals also damage brain cells, contributing to senility and Alzheimer's disease.

DNA
The molecules that program the function and behavior of every cell, sometimes called the blueprint of life.

Although our evolutionary ancestors might have been able to get enough antioxidants from food alone, unfortunately we can't. Saddled with a toxic burden of pesticides, industrial chemicals, pollutants, and a whole witches' brew of toxins in our indoor and outdoor environment, we need antioxidant supplements to protect and nourish the brain.

Antioxidant Nutrients Equal Less Rust

Fortunately, a number of nutrients, including vitamins C and E, reduce the tendency for excess free radicals to be formed and for free-radical damage (including lipid peroxidation) to get out of control.

Lipid Peroxidation
A form of free-radical damage that affects fats, such as the membranes of cells.

How do antioxidants do their thing? First, consider that pro-oxidants are compounds that get in the way of normal metabolism by stealing electrons from, or oxidizing, normal cell macromolecules. If the normal macromolecule affected is DNA, the result can be what's called a mutation. If the normal macromolecule affected is an enzyme, the result can be the shutdown of that enzyme activity.

To protect us against a whole variety of free radicals, we need an array of protective mechanisms with broad defensive powers. Two key antioxidant enzymes are superoxide dismutase and glutathione peroxidase. Together, they work to keep superoxide anion and hydrogen peroxide levels low so that the destructive hydroxyl free radical is not formed. Vitamin C protects us against oxygen-centered free radicals and also restores vitamin E, if oxidized, to its beneficial form. If vitamin C is, in turn, oxidized, it can be restored by selenium-containing glutathione peroxidase. Alpha lipoic acid is able to restore vitamins C and E and to protect glutathione.

Antioxidants, then, are dependent upon each other to function and protect optimally. Thus it's clear that proper levels of antioxidants must be maintained at all times within the complex interrelationships and interdependencies of what is sometimes called the antioxidant network.

Studies show that if your body becomes overwhelmed by free radicals, or if you're not getting enough antioxidant-rich vitamins and minerals from your diet, antioxidant supplements can protect against this free-radical-caused oxidative damage by scavenging, or quenching, free radicals.

If Antioxidants Help Old *Dogs* Learn New Tricks, Then . . .

As in humans, the brains of old dogs accumulate unhealthy deposits of beta-amyloid protein and experience oxidative damage. In humans, the buildup of these protein fragments in the brain's vessels and neurofibrillary tangles (bunched-up neural cells) has been tied to the progression of Alzheimer's disease. In fact, it has been shown that excess free radicals speed up the buildup of beta-amyloid plaque.

Beta-Amyloid Plaque
A hallmark of Alzheimer's disease are deposits in certain regions of the brain of a waxy plaque called beta-amyloid.

Well, now it seems that old dogs truly *can* learn new tricks if given the right levels of antioxidants, according to two studies from 2002.

In one study from the Institute for Brain Aging and Dementia at the University of California's Gillespie Neuroscience Research Facility, researchers gave some old dogs an antioxidant-fortified diet and other dogs standard chow. Dogs that received the antioxidant-rich food had a significantly greater ability to learn new tricks—or, as the researchers put it, "to acquire progressively more difficult learning tasks"—than did the dogs receiving the regular food. In short, the dogs on the enriched diet learned more quickly and better than did their counterparts on standard chow. The study shows, say the authors, that oxidative (free radical) damage impairs mental (cognitive) function and that "antioxidant treatment can result in significant improvements."

In another study, this one from the University of Toronto, researchers looked at antioxidant-fortified chow and how well beagles could learn and remember their surroundings, and locate and remember targets, in what's called a landmark discrimination learning test. The results? In a series of four experiments, the study showed both that oxidative damage causes age-associated cognitive problems and that antioxidant-supplemented food can partially *reverse* aging's normal effects on mental function (cognition).

Clearly, antioxidant compounds help shield mammals—beagles and humans alike—from many of the degenerative brain changes that, if left unchecked, typically accompany aging.

Antioxidant Supplements: Multivitamins

Since you've read this far, or have picked up this book and turned to this page, you've no doubt heard about the world-shaking two-part review paper by Harvard researchers Kathleen M. Fairfield, M.D., and Robert H. Fletcher, M.D., in the July 19, 2002, issue of the *Journal of the American Medical Association,* in which most adult Americans are urged to take a multivitamin in order to ensure adequate dietary levels of vitamins A, B_6, B_{12}, folic acid, and vitamins C and E.

Certainly the two-part article was not earth-shattering to all of us, the supplement savants—we've known this for years. Still, it was a significant admission, on the part of the "Medical Establishment," that dietary supplements are absolutely critical for health.

In fact, back in 1965, J. I. Rodale, the visionary founder of the Rodale Institute and *Prevention* magazine, provided the following insight in his now classic tome, *The Complete Book of Vitamins:*

> It is unfortunate that the effect of poor nutrition on mentality is not more widely publicized. Americans are aware that insufficient rest, sudden shock and certain types of injury can cause mental illness, but the danger to mentality of poor nutrition is one of the better kept secrets of modern research.
>
> Not anymore—it is a secret no longer.

Antioxidant Supplements: Vitamin C

The good news for most mammals is that they can synthesize ascorbic acid, or vitamin C, in their livers. The bad news for Indian fruit bats and humans is that we can't—we are two of several species that need to obtain this essential vitamin from food and, in the case of humans who follow the nutrient-challenged "standard American diet," from dietary supplements. Essential for the growth and repair of tissues in all systems and regions of the body, vitamin C is required for the formation of collagen, connective tissue, bones, and cartilage and is a key powerhouse player in your body's immunity.

Research

Although much of the most recent research on vitamin C has combined this water-soluble nutrient with other vitamins, such as vitamin E, two studies from 1998 show the mind-boosting benefits of vitamin C, how it helps us when it's supplemented, and symptoms that we can experience when it's not.

To test whether vitamin C protects against mental decline, called "cognitive impairment" in this study, researchers from Australia's University of Sydney looked at 117 elderly people in a retirement community over a four-year period—those who took vitamin C supplements and those who did not. What did they find? Seniors who took vitamin C supplements experienced a lower incidence of severe cognitive decline. The authors conclude, "Vitamin C might protect against cognitive impairment."

For all those supplement skeptics and nutritional naysayers who claim that all we need is found in food, French doctors examined vitamin C levels in patients with severe symptoms of

Alzheimer's disease, moderate symptoms of Alzheimer's, and no symptoms. The researchers found that blood levels of vitamin C were significantly lower in patients with Alzheimer's disease compared to the non-Alzheimer's group in "proportion to the degree of cognitive impairment," not explained by vitamin C levels in the diet. In other words, in groups of French people whose symptoms of Alzheimer's disease ranged from none up to severe, the worse the case of Alzheimer's, the lower the blood levels of vitamin C—regardless of the levels of this nutrient consumed in food.

These studies clearly suggest that aggressive supplementation with antioxidants, in this case vitamin C, may be part of a nutritional defense against this devastating disease.

Vitamin C in the Diet

Although there are foods with good concentrations of vitamin C—broccoli, Brussels sprouts, guava, kale, papaya, parsley, spinach, and strawberries, for example—food processing, storage, and exposure to oxygen easily decrease, or eliminate, the vitamin C that was originally present in these sources.

Supplements—How to Choose

Dietary supplements of vitamin C are normally offered as ascorbic acid and as mineral ascorbates. We recommend that you choose vitamin C supplements that also contain bioflavonoids, which are very biologically active natural plant pigments such as quercetin, rutin, hesperidin, and others; these natural plant chemicals improve vitamin C absorption.

Supplements—How to Take and How Much

For vitamin C, what I (SL) call your Optimum Daily

Intake, or ODI (the levels of a nutrient or other dietary supplement needed to help us achieve best possible health, not just to avoid deficiency diseases such as scurvy or beriberi), adult dosage should be between 500 mg and 5,000 mg a day. Many people shoot for 1,000–3,000 mg/day, with 1,000 mg at each meal. If you find that you experience diarrhea once you reach a certain level, then scale back to a dosage range just below this bowel tolerance level, which differs from person to person.

Antioxidant Supplements: Vitamin E

A frequent comrade-at-arms with vitamin C, vitamin E was discovered more than seventy years ago to be a fat-soluble vitamin required for the prevention of fetal death in rats that had been fed a diet of rancid lard.

Vitamin E is really a collection of eight natural forms that occur in one of two groups: tocopherols and tocotrienols (alpha, beta, gamma, and delta forms for each group). Of all the forms of this vitamin, it appears that the only one maintained in our blood plasma is alpha-tocopherol, which is thought to be the most important form of vitamin E and is normally written as d-alpha-tocopherol (or RRR-alpha-tocopherol). Synthetic vitamin E, which can have as little as one-eighth the biological activity of natural vitamin E, is designated as dl-alpha-tocopherol (or all-racemic alpha-tocopherol). Present in cell membranes and the major fat-soluble antioxidant found in blood, red blood cells, and tissues, vitamin E protects your body's cells from free-radical-caused damage.

Research

Two studies from 2002, from as far apart as Chicago and Tokyo, one in humans and the other in rats, set about to determine whether low vitamin E levels were associated with cognitive decline and whether supplementation with this vitamin was effective in combating it.

The Chicago study, which was led by M. C. Morris at the Rush Institute for Healthy Aging, looked at 2,889 community residents, aged 65 to 102 years, from 1993 through 2000. In the group of patients who had the highest level of vitamin E intake, there was a 36 percent reduction in the rate of cognitive decline versus those who had the lowest level of intake. The authors concluded: "Vitamin E intake . . . is associated with less cognitive decline with age."

In the Tokyo study, researchers from Japan's Shibaura Institute of Technology assessed the effects of vitamin E supplementation in rats that experienced oxidative stress and were tested by various learning and memory mazes. The result? Vitamin E supplementation "significantly accelerated" the rats' learning functions and prevented stress-caused memory loss.

Vitamin E in the Diet

Unprocessed vegetable oils are, theoretically, a good source of vitamin E, with corn, soybean, safflower, and wheat germ oils ranking higher in this vitamin than others. Lower concentrations of vitamin E can be found in dark green leafy veggies, nuts, and whole grains. In any case, however, grain milling, food processing, and cooking eliminate virtually all the naturally occurring levels of this vitamin.

Supplements—How to Choose

We recommend that you look for vitamin E succinate and d-alpha-tocopherol with mixed tocopherols (different components of vitamin E, such as alpha-, beta-, delta-, and gamma-tocopherol).

Supplements—How to Take and How Much

For vitamin E, the Optimum Daily Intake to improve mental functioning should be between 400 and 800 IU per day, preferably with a meal. If you have low blood pressure or are taking blood-thinning medications (including aspirin), consult with your licensed healthcare practitioner before taking supplemental vitamin E.

Antioxidant Supplements: Vitamins C and E Combined

Research shows that vitamins C and E work synergistically—that is, when they work together, their biological activity is greater than the sum of their individual benefits. Vitamin E scavenges dangerous free radicals in cell membranes while vitamin C attacks free radicals in biological fluids; in these ways, and others, vitamins C and E reinforce each other's antioxidant effects. Alpha lipoic acid helps both vitamins—but wait: We'll get to alpha lipoic acid in a later chapter.

Research

The April 2003 issue of the *American Journal of Clinical Nutrition* included a study by Harvard's Walter C. Willett, along with two colleagues of his from the Channing Laboratory, on high-dose combination antioxidant supplements (of vitamins C and E) and cognitive function.

The researchers started with data from 14,968 women who originally participated in the Nurses' Health Study. Then, from 1995 to 2000, telephone tests of cognitive function, immediate- and delayed-recall tests, verbal fluency tests, and other tests were administered to these women, who were seventy to seventy-nine years of age at this time.

The findings were powerful indeed: Long-term users of vitamin E with vitamin C scored significantly better on cognitive tests than did women who had never used these vitamins. The benefits were greatest in women who supplemented for the longest periods of time and in women who had the lowest levels of vitamin E from food at the start of the study.

A 2002 study that appeared in the *Journal of the American Medical Association* looked at 5,395 people who were at least fifty-five years of age, free of dementia, and noninstitutionalized at the outset of the study, which ran from 1990 to 1999. It was found that high intake of vitamins C and E was associated with a lower risk for Alzheimer's disease.

Also in 2002, USDA researchers at Tufts University in Boston reviewed the published literature on supplementation with vitamins C and E. They found that these nutrients may improve brain performance and decrease the risk of experiencing age-related mental decline.

Two years before this review, the same research team fortified rat diets with vitamins C and E or a placebo. The high-dose vitamin regimen had positive effects on the brain tissue of these animals and improved the levels of beneficial neurohormones such as dopamine, suggesting, say the researchers, that antioxidants from diet and supplements are critical for brain function.

The same year, an important study on these vitamins was published in the journal *Neurology*. This study, which was part of the Honolulu-Asia Aging Study, has been following 3,385 Japanese American men, aged seventy-one through ninety-three years, whose intake of vitamins C and E had been recorded previously. The results were nothing short of outstanding. A "significant protective effect" was found for vitamins C and E against vascular dementia and other dementias, although not Alzheimer's disease in this particular study. In those without dementia, supplementation with these vitamins was associated with significantly better scores on cognitive tests.

Vascular Dementia
The second most common form of dementia after Alzheimer's disease, vascular dementia is related to circulatory problems and stroke, and is preventable.

The authors conclude that supplements of "vitamins C and E may protect against vascular dementia and may improve cognitive function in late life."

CHAPTER 3

B VITAMINS

Although it often seems a Sisyphean struggle to convince the "Medical Establishment" that targeted nutrients are vital for optimal mental functioning, the B-complex vitamins are an exception, having been accepted for years by many in the stethoscope set as important for cognition. B vitamins are used as coenzymes (important components of enzymes) in almost every area of the body. They are critical for healthy nerves, skin, hair, and vision; they also give us energy since they're needed for the metabolism of carbs, fats, and proteins. Of note, the elderly in particular need supplemental B vitamins since these nutrients are not well absorbed, or metabolized, as we get older.

> **Coenzymes**
> *Vitamins, vitamin-like compounds, or even minerals that aid enzymes in the processing of carbohydrates, fats, and proteins.*

The Bs' well-documented role in nervous system function has even led to many practitioners using therapeutic doses in order to lessen psychiatric symptoms such as mild depression, anxiety, nervousness, and—you guessed it—poor memory.

> **Metabolism**
> *The building-up (anabolic) and breaking-down (catabolic) biochemical reactions and processes in the body.*

In fact, in 1995, Dr. David Benton of the United Kingdom gave ten times the recommended daily allowance of nine vitamins (mostly B complex) to healthy college students for one year. There was a significant improvement in cognitive functioning, especially concentration.

Although the Bs function best when taken as a B-complex supplement, as opposed to taking a handful of individual B vitamins, we'll look at some of the latest research on both combinations and individual B vitamins.

B-Vitamin Roundup

Here's a quick summary of several B vitamins:

- **Thiamine** (vitamin B_1) works as a coenzyme in the metabolism of carbohydrates and branched-chain amino acids; deficiency has been tied to short-term memory decreases, apathy, and confusion. The cells of the brain and nervous system, which are extremely sensitive to carbohydrate metabolism, are the first to show signs of thiamine deficiency. Food sources include organ meats (especially liver), pork, soybeans, brown rice, wheat germ, egg yolks, poultry, and fish. Cooking, as well as exposure to preservatives such as nitrites, destroys a great deal of the thiamine that appears in the food supply. We recommend a B complex, or total supplementation including the B-complex amount (if less than this), of 100–500 mg/day.

- **Riboflavin** (vitamin B_2) functions as a coenzyme in numerous antioxidant reactions; it's helpful for neurological conditions (including carpal tunnel syndrome and certain psychiatric disorders) and for tissue repair. Deficiency may interfere with the metabolism of vitamin B_6. Food sources include cheese, yogurt, eggs, organ meats, poultry, fish, beans, and spinach. Pasteurization, light, and cooking, however, destroy this vitamin rather easily. We recommend a B complex, or total supplementation including the B-complex amount (if less than this), of 100–400 mg/day.

- **Niacin** (vitamin B_3) functions as a coenzyme in many antioxidant reactions; deficiency has been connected to memory loss, anxiety, nervousness, headaches, fatigue, apathy, and depression. Food sources include beef, pork, fish, milk, cheese, whole wheat, potatoes, corn, eggs, broccoli, tomatoes, and carrots; this vitamin is often lost in cooking water. We recommend a B complex, or total supplementation using either a "flush-free" or an extended-release form including the B-complex dose (if less than this), of 100–500 mg/day. If you have any liver problems, please check with your physician before taking high-dose niacin.

- **Vitamin B_6** (pyridoxine) works as a coenzyme in the metabolism, or synthesis, of amino acids, glycogen, and brain proteins; deficiency has been associated with confusion and depression. Food sources include eggs, spinach, carrots, peas, meat, chicken, fish, brewer's yeast, walnuts, sunflower seeds, and wheat germ. In addition to the negative impact of cooking, processing, and refining on this vitamin, the body's ability to use B_6 from foods is very limited. We recommend a B complex, or total supplementation including the B-complex amount (if less than this), of 100–500 mg/day.

- **Folic acid** functions as a coenzyme in specific cases in the metabolism of nucleic and amino acids; deficiency has been linked to difficulty concentrating, depression, schizophrenia, and dementia. Food sources include beef, lamb liver, pork liver, chicken liver, spinach, kale, beet greens, asparagus, broccoli, whole wheat, and brewer's yeast. The body's ability to make use of this vitamin from food is limited, though; in addition, cooking and processing can reduce folic acid content by up to 90 percent. We recommend a B complex, or total supplementation including the B-complex amount (if less than this), of 400–800 mcg/day.

- **Vitamin B$_{12}$** (cobalamin) functions as a coenzyme in the metabolism of fatty acids and in the production of myelin, the fatty substance that covers and protects our nerves; deficiency has been connected to neurological problems (tingling, numbness in extremities), difficulty concentrating, memory loss, mental disorientation, and dementia—specifically Alzheimer's disease. B$_{12}$ levels in food are low to begin with. The sources that do exist include lamb, beef, calf, and pork livers; lamb and beef kidneys; herring; and mackerel. Storage, cooking, and light greatly compromise the integrity of this fragile B vitamin. We recommend a B complex, or total supplementation including the B-complex amount (if less than this), of 100–500 mcg/day.

- **Pantothenic acid** functions as a component of coenzyme A and phosphopantetheine, which are both involved in fatty acid metabolism; deficiency has been tied to apathy, malaise, sleep disturbances, and irritability. Food sources include eggs, potatoes, saltwater fish, pork, beef, milk, whole wheat, peas, beans, and fresh vegetables. A great deal of this vitamin is lost when foods containing pantothenic acid are canned, cooked, frozen, or otherwise processed. We recommend a B complex, or total supplementation including the B-complex amount (if less than this), of 100–500 mg/day. When supplementing with pantothenic acid, make sure that you take sufficient biotin, since these vitamins compete with each other for absorption.

- **Biotin** functions as a coenzyme; deficiency has been tied to depression, lethargy, and hallucinations. Food sources include chicken, lamb, pork, beef, veal, liver, brewer's yeast, soybeans, milk, cheese, saltwater fish, whole-wheat flour, and rice bran. We recommend a B complex, or total supplementation including the B-complex amount (if less than this), of 300–600 mcg/day. When supplementing with biotin, make sure that you take sufficient pantothenic acid, since these vitamins compete with each other for absorption.

- **Choline** functions as a precursor (earlier version) of acetylcholine and phospholipids and is critical for brain transmission; deficiency has been linked to dementia. Food sources include legumes, organ and muscle meats, milk, whole-grain cereals, and egg yolk. We recommend a B complex, or total supplementation including the B-complex amount (if less than this), of 250–500 mg/day.

B-Vitamin Research

In the March–April 2003 edition of the *American Journal of Geriatric Psychiatry*, researchers looked at sixty-nine people with Alzheimer's disease, including thirty-three patients who were taking a multivitamin supplement of folic acid, vitamin B_6, and vitamin B_{12}.

In the sixty-six patients who were available for the eight-week follow-up, the high-dose B-vitamin supplement significantly reduced levels of homocysteine, which is important since high levels of homocysteine may be associated with the breakdown of the myelin sheaths that encase nerves and may be partly responsible for the symptoms of Alzheimer's-like dementia. In addition, the vascular and circulatory problems that often accompany Alzheimer's, such as atherosclerosis (which contributes to the "hardening of the arteries" associated with dementia and cardiovascular disease), owe part of their development to sustained high levels of homocysteine in the blood over time.

Homocysteine
A normal breakdown product of the essential amino acid methionine. At high levels, however, homocysteine causes or contributes to Alzheimer's disease, atherosclerosis, and other conditions.

Australian researchers, in 2002, set out to measure the effects of folic acid (750 mcg/day), vitamin B_6 (75 mg/day), and vitamin B_{12} (15 mcg/day) or a placebo on cognition in 211 healthy younger, middle-aged, and older women. Results? Supplementation, say the authors, had a "significant positive effect on . . . measures of memory performance," and also improved mental (speed) processing, recall, recognition, and verbal ability.

In 2001, Dutch scientists found a prevalence of low levels of vitamin B_{12} in a population-based group of 698 older adults, which the researchers correlated with slower thinking ("reduced information processing speed") compared to participants with normal B_{12} levels.

The same year, Swedish neuroscientists reported their findings relating to 101 elderly patients who were being seen for mental function concerns referred to as "cognitive disturbances" by these researchers. Of the 101 patients, 57 had full-blown dementia (Alzheimer's disease or vascular) and 32 had more mild symptoms.

After examining samples of cerebrospinal fluid and blood from the patients, the researchers saw that decreasingly low levels of cerebrospinal fluid vitamin B_{12}, in addition to increasingly low blood levels of folic acid and B_{12} and increasingly high levels of homocysteine, were associated with escalating degrees of mental, or cognitive, impairment.

Atherosclerosis
In this, the most common form of arteriosclerosis, fatty deposits (plaque) collect on the interior of artery walls.

Earlier the same year, another group of Swedish researchers looked at supplementation with B_{12} and folic acid in thirty-three elderly patients with dementia. Supplemented patients who had mild to moderate dementia and elevated homocysteine levels improved mentally, according to the results of what is referred to as a Mini-Mental State Examination (MMSE). Interestingly, people who had severe dementia and normal homocysteine levels did not appear to respond to the nutritional intervention.

Yet another European group of scientific investigators published their results that year using B_{12} in older people. In this placebo-controlled study, sixteen healthy elderly subjects with low blood levels of vitamin B_{12} and no overt cognitive problems received this vitamin for five months. Before and after the period of vitamin therapy, cognitive and clinical tests were conducted. After the five-month period of supplementation, the following improvements were noted: better performance on mental tests (such as the Verbal Word Learning Test), higher blood levels of the vitamin, and lower levels of homocysteine. In fact, those who achieved the lowest levels of homocysteine did best on the cognitive assessments. Not only that: The cognitive improvements were also seen by comparing before-and-after brain scans that were focused on cerebral function!

An earlier study, this from 2000, looked at vitamin levels and cognitive function in Medicare patients in Bernalillo County, New Mexico. After adjusting for supplement use and a variety of other factors, the researchers found that the elderly people who did poorest on cognitive tests were those who had the lowest levels of folic acid in their blood, with lesser associations tied to levels of vitamins B_{12} and C.

Fast-forwarding to more recent findings, Dr. Alan L. Miller wrote in a 2003 review that patients who respond best to B-vitamin supplementation "appear to be those with mild-to-moderate dementia." He goes on to say: "Since B_{12}, folic acid . . . and vitamin B_6 have been proven to lower homocysteine levels and are an inexpensive preventive measure, supplementation is a prudent preventive choice in middle-aged to elderly individuals."

CHAPTER 4

ALPHA LIPOIC ACID AND ACETYL-L-CARNITINE

A lpha what? That's what I (JG) said before April 1996, when the secretariats of the United Nations and the World Health Organization (WHO) convened the groundbreaking First Joint Conference on Healthy Ageing.

Some of the most exciting findings presented at the summit focused on alpha lipoic acid (ALA), a vitaminlike compound that has been found to directly restore vitamin C and glutathione to their active antioxidative forms after they have been used up, and to indirectly restore vitamin E to its active form after it has been depleted. It also can increase levels of coenzyme Q_{10} in our cells.

Alpha lipoic acid is also a very powerful antioxidant in its own right. In fact, ALA can operate in both watery and fatty areas of the body and can, therefore, protect all parts of the cells of the body from free radical damage.

According to the *Physicians' Desk Reference (PDR) for Nutritional Supplements*, animal studies are "suggestive of some . . . benefit from lipoic acid in the treatment of various neurodegenerative disorders, including . . . Alzheimer's disease."

Acetyl-L-carnitine (ALC) is another vitaminlike nutrient, and is related in structure to the B vitamins. L-carnitine may also be important for healthy brain function since it appears to beneficially influence the metabolism of several neurotransmitters; it also has antioxidant powers in its own right.

Acetyl-L-carnitine is another form of L-carnitine that is believed to "have neuroprotective effects," according to the *PDR for Nutritional Supplements*. A significant body of accumulating research points to acetyl-L-carnitine's beneficial effects in Alzheimer's patients, especially in regard to attention and concentration. There is also evidence, says the *PDR*, that "acetyl-L-carnitine can slow mental decline" in older people who do not have dementia.

> **Neurotransmitter**
> A chemical, such as dopamine, acetylcholine, norepinephrine, or serotonin, that influences brain or nervous system activity.

According to a review by Dr. Parris Kidd, acetyl-L-carnitine is "an energizer and metabolic co-factor which also benefits various cognitive functions in the middle-aged and elderly."

The More, the Merrier

If one brain-boosting nutrient is good, could more be better? Sometimes the answer is a resounding yes. An affirmative was certainly a conclusion arrived at by doctors at Leipzig's Interdisciplinary Center for Clinical Research in a study that appeared in the February 2003 edition of the *Journal of Alzheimer's Disease*.

In a series of test-tube experiments, these German researchers started out with a recognition that advanced glycation end-products (AGEs)—sugar-derived modified proteins and products of lipid peroxidation—are prominent features of Alzheimer's disease. It's already known that AGE "gunk" builds up in the brains of people with Alzheimer's disease.

The researchers looked at human brain cells and conditions that mimic these free-radical and plaque-accumulation ("gunking up") changes that normally occur with Alzheimer's disease. Demonstrating a direct biochemical link between AGEs and lipid peroxidation, the authors point out that using specific antioxidants that fight AGEs, such as alpha lipoic acid, N-acetylcysteine, and others, showed less formation of AGE gunk and byproducts of free-radical assault. The authors speculate that these cognition-boosting supplements could also help protect the human brain from the changes that occur in aging and Alzheimer's disease.

Three thousand miles away, researchers at the Geriatric Research Education and Clinical Center in St. Louis, Missouri, started their animal study with an acknowledgment that free-radical-caused bombardment (also called oxidative stress) may "play a crucial role in age-related neurodegenerative disorders."

In a strain of mice especially prone to age-related neurological changes (which appear as early as twelve months of age), supplementation with alpha lipoic acid and N-acetylcysteine improved cognition (learning, memory) in these twelve-month-old rodents. According to the authors, "these results support the [recognition] that oxidative stress can lead to cognitive dysfunction and provide evidence for a therapeutic role for antioxidants."

Enter Alpha Lipoic Acid and Acetyl-L-Carnitine . . .

A year before, in 2002, a team of scientists at the University of California–Berkeley, led by Dr. Bruce Ames, began their animal-model experiments with the understanding that decay of our cells' energy factories, mitochondria, occurs in normal aging, not just Alzheimer's.

In a group of old rats, supplementing with acetyl-L-carnitine and alpha lipoic acid improved age-associated declines in memory and, in fact, protected brain cells themselves from some of the free radical damage and changes normally brought on by aging. Bottom line? Age-related mitochondrial decay "can be reversed"—yes, *reversed*—through supplementation with acetyl-L-carnitine and alpha lipoic acid.

Also in 2002, at the prestigious Linus Pauling Institute in Corvallis, Oregon, researchers, in this case again led by Bruce Ames, found that administering chow supplemented with alpha lipoic acid and acetyl-L-carnitine to young and old rats improved a number of measures associated with healthy brain aging and overall aging. Rats had better energy levels and even moved around better, to boot.

Now let's take a deeper look at the research on these nutrients that seems to be currently—in the mind-boosting area, at least—weighted in favor of acetyl-L-carnitine.

Acetyl-L-Carnitine

A 2003 meta-analysis from London's Imperial College University looked at acetyl-L-carnitine in cases of mild cognitive impairment and "mild" Alzheimer's disease in parallel three-month, six-month, and twelve-month studies.

Results? A "significant advantage" for the participants treated with acetyl-L-carnitine versus those who received the look-alike placebo. Beneficial effects were seen by three months in patients with either mild cognitive impairment or mild Alzheimer's disease; interestingly, the benefits appeared to be cumulative since they increased over time.

Although a number of animal-model and test-tube studies using acetyl-L-carnitine came out between 1999 and 2003, the next most compelling human study was published in 1998 by Stanford University researchers led by Dr. John Brooks. This trial involved twenty-four clinical centers and 334 people diagnosed with "probable Alzheimer's disease."

Interestingly, the younger patients treated with ALC—those aged sixty-one and under—experienced a significantly slower mental decline, or progression of Alzheimer's disease, than did patients who received the placebo. In fact, the authors write, "ALC slows the progression of Alzheimer's disease in younger patients." Then what's stopping you and us from taking it as a preventive?

Two years previous to this, a group of neuroscientists at the UCSD School of Medicine in La Jolla, California, looked at acetyl-L-carnitine in patients with what was referred to as "probable Alzheimer's disease." In this study, 357 people with mild-to-moderate Alzheimer's disease, aged fifty and older, completed one year on a regimen that included either 3,000 mg/day of ALC or a placebo. Using two major rating systems, the Alzheimer's Disease Assessment Scale and the Clinical Dementia Rating Scale, the most mental benefits (that is, the slowest decline) were again seen in the relatively younger subset of patients, those aged sixty-five and younger.

What about just mental function as we get older, not Alzheimer's disease? Well, a 1994 study out of Modena, Italy, examined 481 people and ALC spread out over forty-four different clinical centers over 150 days. The cognitive improvements alone with ALC were extremely significant, with a p value of less than 0.0001—a statistical power that is enough to make an actuary blush.

Not only that, but clinical measures of memory, emotion, stress, and mood also markedly improved. Therefore, this study showed that acetyl-L-carnitine also helps the "mild mental impairment" that many people develop as they pass the middle-aged period.

Alpha Lipoic Acid

In 2001, researchers gave eight men and one woman with primary degenerative dementia (Alzheimer's disease), aged fifty-two through eighty-one years, 600 mg/day of alpha lipoic acid in addition to an acetylcholinesterase inhibitor (Aricept or Exelon) for up to three years. Due to the significant stabilizing of mental function over and above typical drug-only results, the authors conclude that "alpha-lipoic acid may be a neuroprotective" supplement.

The same year, the National Institute of Mental Health (part of the National Institutes of Health, or NIH) wanted to see what would happen if they treated rat brain cells (cortical neurons), which in rats and humans are prone to the aging-related accumulation of beta-amyloid plaque, with alpha lipoic acid, an antioxidant considered "an ideal substance" for this application by these NIH behavioral endocrinologists.

Endocrinologist
A physician who specializes in glands that secrete directly into the bloodstream, including the pituitary gland, pancreas, thyroid, and adrenal gland.

The United States government researchers found that treatment with ALA protected brain cells against both plaque and free radical attack, providing even more backup for alpha lipoic's neuroprotective benefits.

Back in 1993, researchers administered alpha lipoic to old female mice. The results were clear:

ALA reduced age-related decline and improved memory, probably due, speculate the researchers, to the potent antioxidant protection that the nutrient provided to these aging animals.

Supplements—How to Take and How Much

- **Acetyl-L-carnitine:** Typical doses of supplemental acetyl-L-carnitine are 500–2,000 mg/day in divided doses.

- **Alpha lipoic acid:** Typical doses are 100–600 mg/day (600–1,200 mg for Alzheimer's disease) in divided doses; people with diabetes should monitor their blood glucose levels while supplementing with ALA since their physician may need to lower their doses of antidiabetic medications.

CHAPTER 5

HERBS

A friend of ours, James A. Duke, Ph.D., has nearly thirty-five years of experience working with medicinal herbs—from the jungles of Latin America to the research labs of the United States Department of Agriculture (USDA), from which he retired as chief ethnobotanist and the world's undisputed authority on medicinal herbs. If he is convinced that herbs and herbal supplements offer benefits for the mind, who are we to argue?

Perhaps ironically after all this time, only several years ago Dr. Duke started taking ginkgo (*Ginkgo biloba*) after he read a study in the *Journal of the American Medical Association* that "acknowledged," he said, "that ginkgo might help slow the effects of old age on the brain, which they called senile dementia."

Senile Dementia
A chronic mental disease of late life that typically gets progressively worse and is marked by failing memory and decline of cognitive/ intellectual functions.

Duke says, "Senile dementia is a blanket term for getting addled in your old age, and it includes Alzheimer's disease." When asked, "Why are you taking ginkgo?" Duke wrote, characteristically: "I'm taking ginkgo as a preventive, not for anything chronic. One doesn't notice any changes when one prevents something, and so far, I'd say the ginkgo is doing its job."

The Science Behind Brain-Boosting Herbs

Fortunately, there are many published scientific studies that provide evidence supporting not only ginkgo's cognition-boosting benefits but also those of ginseng, alone and in combination with ginkgo. There are also findings that support the use of gotu kola and specialized plant-derived extracts (such as vinpocetine, which we'll get to in the next chapter).

In traditional Chinese medicine, ginseng (*Panax ginseng*) has been one of the few herbs that is used by itself on a daily basis as a "health and longevity tonic." In the same tradition, an extract of the leaves of gotu kola (*Centella asiatica*) has been indicated to boost energy and mental function; both of these botanicals are considered antiaging tonics.

Ginkgo and Friends

Often called a living fossil, the ginkgo trees that line city sidewalks today are, for all intents and purposes, the same trees that shaded dinosaurs 100 to 200 million years ago, a time that spanned both the Cretaceous and Jurassic periods. *Ginkgo biloba* is so old, writes Duke, "that it once grew widely throughout the northern hemisphere at a time when lands bordering the Arctic Ocean were warm and balmy."

Over the last few decades, a great deal of research on this herb has been building. According to *Herbal Medicine—Expanded Commission E Monographs* (2000), there have been "over 400 scientific studies conducted on proprietary standardized extracts of the leaf of ginkgo in the past 30 years."

Ginseng, on the other hand, is native to the mountain forests of northeastern China and the far eastern reaches of Russia. Wild ginseng is now banned for harvest and trade by both Russia and China. In China, Korea, and Japan, ginseng today comes from cultivated sources. According to *Herbal Medicine,* ginseng's therapeutic uses were recorded in one of the world's oldest known comprehensive medical references, the *Shen Nongh Ben Cao Jing,* which was written about 2,000 years ago. Legend has it that Chinese warlords would kill peasants who tried to steal ginseng during harvest. To this day, the value of certain types of ginseng root is such that they cost as much as an ounce of gold—and I know this because I used to sell it on the Home Shopping Network (SL)!

Ginseng was traditionally used "as an aid during convalescence and as a [preventive] to build resistance, reduce susceptibility to illness and promote health and longevity." It was most certainly not used, however, as an herbal version of a Starbucks grande with an extra shot.

Giving Credit Where Credit Is Due . . .

In poring through the research, we uncovered the fact that a lion's share of the research on ginkgo has been carried out on a ginkgo extract, EGb 761, which is sold as Ginkgold and Ginkgold Max by Nature's Way in the United States. Another ginkgo product that has been well researched is GK501, or more popularly Ginkoba and Ginkoba Mental Endurance (a combination of ginkgo and ginseng) sold by Pharmaton in the United States; much of the research on ginseng was also carried out by Pharmaton, which produces G115, an extract sold as Ginsana in the United States.

Ginkgo and Ginseng Together

As is the case with other carefully balanced

herbal combination remedies (or recipes) in China, Tibet, and India, as well as Native American nations (interestingly, the Menominee tribe used ginseng as a mental tonic), studies have uncovered that, although ginkgo and ginseng are each powerful mind boosters by themselves, the *combination* of ginkgo and ginseng appears to produce significant synergistic benefits—meaning that the sum of the two is more powerful than each herb alone.

Synergy
The phenomenon seen when factors (in this case, herbs) taken in combination produce results that exceed the sum of the individual results when each factor is taken separately.

In a 2002 issue of *Human Psychopharmacology*, researchers from England's University of Northumbria published their results of three studies designed to look at single doses of ginkgo (GK501, or Ginkoba), ginseng (G115, or Ginsana), and their combination in healthy young people (with a mean age of twenty-one years) during arithmetic tests of varying difficulty ("with differing cognitive load"). A number of important improvements were seen with each of the treatments compared to the "dummy pills" or placebo. Specifically, ginkgo alone improved a subject's "speed of responding" to subtraction tasks. Ginseng by itself improved accuracy.

The "most striking results," however, say the authors, came about following a 320 mg supplement dose of the ginkgo-ginseng combination (Ginkoba Mental Endurance). In addition, the higher-dose combination of 640 mg and 960 mg improved accuracy, as well. As to why the combination worked so well for these investigators, they write:

> Medical herbalism emphasizes *synergy* between components of plant extracts. It

would appear that the comprehensive improvements in performance associated with the ginkgo-ginseng combination represent synergistic behavioural effects of the two extracts interacting with cognitive demand.

Later the same year, these British researchers published the results of a study also looking at ginkgo, ginseng, and both, but in this case focusing on the potential effects on mood and cognitive performance. Twenty healthy people received a single dose of ginkgo (360 mg), a single dose of ginseng (400 mg), a combination product with both, or a placebo.

The results? All three treatments were associated with improved (secondary) memory performance, with ginseng more effective at improving the speed of performing memory tasks and the accuracy of "attentional tasks." Based on the results of subtraction tests, cognitive performance was improved with either ginkgo alone or with the combo. Ginkgo by itself also appeared to improve mood.

A still-earlier study (2001) from these same researchers found that the combination of ginkgo and ginseng produced powerful results in a dose-dependent manner—meaning that the 960 mg combination supplement yielded the most dramatic improvements, especially in the area of what scientists call "quality of memory."

Dose-Dependent
Benefits increase in direct correlation with increasing levels (or dosage) of a given herb (vitamin, mineral, drug, or other compound).

Ginkgo

In 2002, New York University (NYU) Medical Center researchers published the results of a fifty-two-week, intent-to-treat double-blind placebo-controlled study using 120 mg/day of ginkgo (Ginkoba) in patients with varying degrees of mental, or cognitive, impairment.

Improvements were observed in measures of cognitive performance and what was termed "social functioning"—being able to satisfactorily communicate and interact with others. The best improvements were seen in those patients with mild cognitive impairment; in people with "more severe dementia" the benefits were more along the lines of stabilizing or slowing down the decline.

The same year, a study using Ginkoba was published that looked at supplementation in a group of sixty-six healthy participants aged fifty through sixty-five years. According to the American Botanical Council's December 31, 2002, *HerbClip*, the subjects used either 240 mg/day of this extract or a placebo daily for four weeks. The findings indicated that "the extract had a beneficial effect on mental performance." Other specific improvements included enhanced motor skills and an "improved sense of well being."

One year earlier, in 2001, the Institute for Natural Products Research in St. Croix, Minnesota, published a review of the ginkgo research out there and concluded: "Clinical studies have shown that ginkgo extracts exhibit therapeutic activity in [many] disorders, including Alzheimer's disease, failing memory, age-related dementias, poor cerebrovascular blood flow," and other conditions.

In Australia, that same year, the *International Journal of Neuropsychopharmacology* described a study in which sixty-one people underwent a gauntlet of cognitive tests both before and after a thirty-day treatment run with ginkgo (or a placebo). Analysis of the results shows that

"significant improvements in speed of information processing" related to memory were achieved
in the ginkgo-supplemented participants.

In 1999, a five-year ginkgo treatment study
(called the Ginkgo Evaluation of Memory trial,
or GEM) funded through the National Center
for Complementary and Alternative Medicine
(NCCAM) was announced by Wake Forest University in Winston-Salem, North Carolina. Involving four sites and geared to enroll 3,000 people
aged seventy-five and older without Alzheimer's
disease, the treatment group received 240 mg of
ginkgo each day. Preliminary results, which were
presented to the NIH on August 23, 2002, are
promising.

Ginseng

In February 2003, at the American Stroke Association's Twenty-eighth International Stroke Conference, a Chinese study by Jinzhou Tian, M.D.,
compared the effects of Chinese ginseng extract
with those of a memory drug (Duxil) in forty
patients with moderate stroke-caused vascular
dementia who were an average age of sixty-
seven.

According to Tian, memory loss, or dementia,
may occur after a stroke and is a growing problem in China. At the start and end of the twelve-
week study, participants took memory tests
focusing on story recall, word recall, verbal learning, verbal recognition, and visual recognition.

Overall, the researchers found that "patients
who took the ginseng compound significantly
improved their average memory function after
twelve weeks," indicating that ginseng appears
to improve memory after a stroke.

An earlier study, in this case in 2001 by the
same group of psychologists from the University

of Northumbria, in England, who carried out the 2002 ginkgo-ginseng combination experiments, looked at the mental-boosting effects of ginseng (G115, or Ginsana) in healthy adults. Twenty "healthy young adults" received 200 mg, 400 mg, or 600 mg of ginseng, or a matching placebo. Following a baseline mental (cognitive) evaluation, people were tested at one, two-and-a-half, four, and six hours after the day's treatment. According to the investigators, the "most striking result" was a significant improvement in "quality of memory" and "secondary memory," or how "good" or detailed the memory function actually was. The ginseng group experienced faster attention speeds, as well.

Other Herbs

Sage

In ancient Egypt, sage (*Salvia officinalis*) was believed to increase fertility in women. Today what is now known as a "kitchen herb" is being studied for its mind-enhancing effects.

In fact, in September 2003 a group of English researchers published their results using sage for memory. Out of a group of forty-four healthy young adults between eighteen and thirty-seven years of age, some were given capsules containing sage oil while others received a placebo capsule. The participants then performed a word-recall test. The results? Those who took the sage oil did "consistently better" than those who took the placebo. Lead researcher Nicola Tildesley said: "This research has serious implications for Alzheimer's disease."

Gotu Kola

Gotu kola (*Centella asiatica*) was originally used to treat leprosy in Asia. Current practitioners of traditional medicine still use the juice of the leaves for sores. In terms of mind boosting, however, modern research has indeed pointed to this plant's benefits.

In a 2002 Indian study involving rats by M. H. Veerendra Kumar and Y. K. Gupta, treatment with an extract of gotu kola significantly improved measures of learning and memory, leading the researchers to speculate that the use of supplements of this botanical may provide "cognitive enhancing effects."

Supplements—How to Take and How Much

- **Ginkgo:** Take 120–240 mg/day in two to three divided doses; the product should be standardized to 24 percent ginkgolides (also called flavonoid glycosides).

- **Ginseng:** Try 400 mg/day; the product should be standardized to 4 to 8 percent ginsenosides.

- **Sage:** Take 2.5–7.5 g/day of sage tincture or 1.5–3 g of liquid extract (or consider that 1 teaspoon of sage in food is about 1.5 g).

- **Gotu kola:** Try 400–500 mg/day in capsule form; look for products containing a high total percentage of triterpenoids.

CHAPTER 6

SPECIALIZED SUPPLEMENTS

We now want to introduce you to "designer supplements"—supplements that are specialized extracts of, or in some cases several steps away from, growing things in nature, including periwinkle, Chinese club moss, French maritime pine bark, and grapes. These also include supplements with names so cumbersome if they were spelled out that even those who consider themselves "supplement savvy" or among the "capsule cognoscenti" can't easily remember them when pressed. (We use their better-known initials—NADH, DMAE, and others.) Nevertheless, these supplements have benefits—some well established, some for which research is building—that are not, fortunately, easy to forget.

Vinpocetine

Vinpocetine is one such supplement. It's derived from vincamine, an extract of the periwinkle plant (*Vinca minor*), and has been widely used and studied in Europe for more than twenty-five years. Awareness of this product and the research behind it is now starting to come into its own.

Based on the results of animal and human studies, vinpocetine has been recommended as a treatment for stroke in Hungary, Poland, Germany, Russia, and Japan. Its ability to boost brain circulation and how the brain makes use of oxygen is the key finding between 1976—when vinpocetine seems to have been first looked at—and today.

A 2002 review (meta-analysis) in the *Journal of the American Nutraceutical Association* by the University of Miami's Bernd Wollschlaeger, M.D., winnowed down thirty-nine vinpocetine studies involving 1,912 subjects into three studies—from 1986 through 1991—involving a total of 174 patients treated with vinpocetine and 114 given a placebo.

According to Wollschlaeger, all three studies "suggest a significant improvement in the cognitive [mental] function of patients suffering from dementia or other symptoms of cerebrovascular diseases." Based on several mental performance tests, the significant improvement in cognitive function in these three studies, says Wollschlaeger, "suggest[s] a clinical application of vinpocetine in the early phases of mild cognitive impairment" before full-blown senile dementia or Alzheimer's disease start to develop.

Out of Hungary came an earlier review article, in 2001, in which "the beneficial effect[s] of vinpocetine" are linked to its ability to improve brain circulation. In 1990, Japanese researchers found that vinpocetine supplementation improved circulation, including that in the brain, in patients with vascular dementia. Wollschlaeger believes that there truly is a "window of opportunity" between mild cognitive impairment and dementia or Alzheimer's disease. He writes that "the utilization of . . . vinpocetine might slow the disease process and decrease its incidence." In this study, an increase in blood flow and brain circulation was noted after only a single 5 mg dose of vinpocetine.

A 1986 study, in this case out of Venice, Italy,

used 30 mg per day of vinpocetine for thirty days in twenty-two elderly patients with brain-circulatory and neurological impairment. Results? Compared to the placebo group, the patients who were on vinpocetine scored significantly higher in all evaluations, including the Mini-Mental State Examination.

Huperzine A

Huperzine A is a purified substance derived from Chinese club moss (*Huperzia serrata*). Some scientists believe that supplements of huperzine A prevent the breakdown of acetylcholine, an important brain-signal-transmitting chemical. The body's loss of proper acetylcholine function is a key feature of several brain-related conditions, including Alzheimer's disease. It is believed that huperzine A may protect brain tissue, as well.

In fact, a 2002 study that appeared in the journal *Brain Research* looked at the protective effects of this supplement in rats. In an experiment designed to mirror the kinds of deterioration that can occur in the human brain when people experience hypoxic-ischemic encephalopathy (in which arterial blood flow to the brain is blocked, and the resulting oxygen deprivation causes brain damage), huperzine A treatment protected against the effects of brain damage and preserved mental function.

The year before, the same lead researcher, X. C. Tang, and a different group of scientists had looked at huperzine A supplementation in gerbils. Again, huperzine A reduced memory loss and brain (neuron) damage after experimentally induced ischemia.

Ischemia
A decrease in, or obstruction of, arterial blood flow.

We looked at beta-amyloid "gunk" earlier in this book, those nasty protein deposits that build up in the brains of people with Alzheimer's disease. Well, in another 2001 study by X. C. Tang, huperzine A reduced the mental (cognitive) changes in rats that had beta-amyloid injected into their brain cavities (cerebral ventricles). The authors concluded that the "beneficial effects" of this supplement suggest that "huperzine A is a promising therapeutic agent for Alzheimer's disease."

In a study with monkeys in 1999, huperzine A "significantly reversed" deterioration of working memory that had been experimentally induced. The authors also found that the supplement improved working memory, suggesting, the researchers say, that "huperzine A may be a promising agent for clinical therapy of cognitive impairments in patients with Alzheimer's disease."

In a 1995 study out of China, 58 percent of patients with Alzheimer's disease experienced "significant improvement in memory" and cognitive and behavioral functions after taking 400 mcg of huperzine A daily for two months.

Pycnogenol and OPCs

Thousands of years ago, naturally occurring free-radical-fighting pigments—bioflavonoids—that occur in plants, fruits, and vegetables, today called oligomeric proanthocyanidins (or OPCs), were extracted from the bark of pine trees growing along the Atlantic by North American Indians and decocted into a tea. In 1534, the French explorer Jacques Cartier was introduced to the tea when Native Americans used it to save most of his crew from death by scurvy during the winter of 1534.

More than 400 years later, a French scientist working in Canada, Jacques Masquelier, was the first to identify and characterize these bioflavonoid compounds as 85 percent oligomeric proanthocyanidins, other compounds, and water. Masquelier developed a process to extract these compounds—both from pine bark (in 1951) and from grape seeds (1970). He used the term *pycnogenol* to refer to this whole family of OPCs.

It is believed that OPCs are very highly concentrated, in a healthful balance, in the bark of these pine trees. Today, Pycnogenol, from French maritime pine, is a multi-patent-protected brand name owned by Horphag Research Ltd., headquartered in Guernsey, in the Channel Islands.

In 2002, a review study that appeared in the *International Journal of Clinical Pharmacology and Therapeutics* found that Pycnogenol is a powerful antioxidant that "improves cognitive function."

Earlier research, from 2000, by Benjamin Lau at Loma Linda University concluded that Pycnogenol "helps to prevent vascular damage in the brain [caused by] beta amyloid [plaque]." In Lau's research, old mice fed with this supplement "showed markedly improved memory and learning ability."

Other Designer Supplements for the Brain

NADH and DMAE are two other supplements for which cognition-focused research is building. *NADH* stands for "reduced beta-nicotinamide adenine dinucleotide with high-energy hydrogen"; also known as coenzyme 1, it's an antioxidant form of vitamin B_3 (niacin). It is thought by some scientists to be the "spark" that ignites energy production in the cells of the body, and is also believed to protect the brain chemical dopamine from a dangerous type of deterioration called auto-oxidation. DMAE, or dimethylamino-ethanol, may increase levels of the brain neuro-transmitter acetylcholine.

A published 2002 study used the patented Enada NADH in a study looking at brain fog produced by jet lag in thirty-five healthy adults who were given either Enada NADH or a placebo after traveling on a red-eye flight from the West Coast to the East Coast of the United States. The findings? People who received Enada NADH "performed significantly better on [four] cognitive test measures" than did their placebo-taking counterparts.

In a 1996 study with 60 elderly patients who reported poor concentration and low performance on cognitive tests, treatment with DMAE successfully reversed certain electrochemical brain changes that were seen on electroencephalogram (EEG) recordings; these improvements were not seen in the placebo group.

Supplements—How to Take and How Much

- **Vinpocetine:** Try 60 mg/day with food; follow label directions.

- **Huperzine A:** Try 50–400 mcg/day in divided doses; follow label directions.

- **Pycnogenol:** Try 150–200 mg/day with or right after meals.

- **NADH:** Try 10 mg/day, with water only, on an empty stomach; follow label directions.

- **DMAE:** Try 100 mg/day; follow label directions.

CHAPTER 7

TRAINING YOUR BRAIN

All of our thoughts and cogitations, memories and musings, dreams and aspirations, pleasures and pains are, as psychologist Ian H. Robertson writes, "embroidered in a trembling web of 100 billion brain cells."

Since, on average, each brain cell is connected 1,000 times with other neurons, we're looking at a web of 100,000 billion connections! It is said that there are more cell synapses (meeting points or regions of communication) in one human brain than there are stars in this galaxy.

Paying attention to a single task, such as reading this sentence, enhances the electrochemical synaptic firing that goes on in the parts of the brain responsible for, in this case, vision and cognition. Right now, the touch- and hearing-oriented areas of your brain are in standby mode since you're not involved in a touching-focused activity, which is why you didn't hear the person in the room calling you just now: You were concentrating your brain's neuronal web on what you were reading.

Paying attention and concentrating can, as Robertson writes, "sculpt brain activity by turning

Neuron
The complete nerve cell, including the cell body, axon, and dendrites.

Synapse
The point at which an impulse passes from an axon of one neuron to a dendrite or to the cell of another.

up or down the rate at which particular sets of synapses fire—and since we know that firing a set of synapses again and again makes the trembling web grow bigger and stronger, it follows that attention is an important ingredient for brain sculpture."

So what does all this mean?

Use it or lose it! And the more you use your brain—consistently over time—the longer you will be able to hold on to it. We may scoff at the seeming obviousness of this: Thinking is good for the brain. But isn't it true that a brain is a brain is a brain? Not necessarily.

In the mid-1980s, Dr. Marian Diamond, then of the Lawrence Hall of Science at the University of California–Berkeley, was chosen to dissect the brain of Albert Einstein and compare it to eleven other brains. The result? Einstein had an enhanced grouping of cells in what is called "Area 39." Area 39 is the most highly evolved part of the brain, a region rich in the glial cells that support the work of thinking neurons as well as what is considered fluid intelligence—a measure of how efficiently the brain works.

Dr. Dharma Singh Khalsa wrote, in 1997, that Einstein's "genius was probably more a result of what he had done with his brain." Dr. Khalsa added, "He had enlarged the most important part of the brain by mentally exercising it to the maximum possible degree—in effect, Einstein was a 'mental athlete' who had 'trained hard' all his life."

Building on Dr. Diamond's discoveries, Seattle's Dr. K. Warner Schaie tracked the cognitive development of people in the Seattle region. By the 1980s, many of the participants in his study had hit what Dr. Khalsa described as the "memory barrier" of their fifties and sixties. They showed dramatic declines in inductive reasoning and spatial orientation—the brain functions that are typically among the first to worsen as we age.

Dr. Schaie offered some of the participants mental "exercise" classes designed to boost inductive reasoning and spatial orientation. Thanks to these cognitive classes, the mental abilities of more than half of the subjects improved greatly.

The Carpe Diem Approach

In 2002, neurologist Jeff Victoroff wrote:

> What, precisely, should you do . . . to help save your brain? Read the encyclopedia? . . . The real answer is to live life to its fullest—not merely watch television and wait for cataracts to blur the image, and not merely exist or occupy space and pass time, [awaiting] the moment when the wristwatch is taken from the wrist. Leap with both feet into the future.

By this, Dr. Victoroff means that we should be seeking out and embracing new things, or, as he puts it, "diving into new seas of neural natation." Active, deliberate learning appears to challenge our neural system—and brain—if it is exciting enough, and enjoyable enough, to regularly and continually keep us motivated and engaged.

The following are some suggestions offered by Dr. Victoroff:

- Care passionately about what you learn and apply it *daily* in a "newly challenging lifestyle."

- Never retire your mind.

- Go back to school.

- Learn a game that you haven't mastered yet.

- Change your career at age fifty.

- Create a Web site.

- Learn to speak a new language.

- Take up a musical instrument you have always wanted to play.

- Create those poems or paint those paintings.

- Travel.

- Compose.

- Invent.

- Teach others.

Is That Mnemonic or Pneumonic? I Don't Recall

Mnemonic

Any conscious pattern or grouping of items, words, or data intended to aid later recollection; any rhyme or other device that aids memory.

Do you remember that trick for recalling the order of the planets? **M**y **V**ery **E**xcellent **M**other **J**ust **S**erved **U**s **N**ine **P**izzas. That is a mnemonic— a trick that helps us remember something, usually something hard to remember, such as a long list.

There are tricks we can do every day to help us remember things better. These are not parlor games but truly ways we can package information and experience so that our brain will be more inclined to stay sharp longer, and so that our memory works better.

Here are some techniques that should help:

- **Anchoring memory to emotion:** Since the norepinephrine released during an emotional experience helps the brain "transport" the recollection of the experience into long-term storage, we know that anchoring things we want to remember to an emotionally charged image often helps. If you are trying to remember directions, for instance, picture your car crashing into a wall (in a cartoonlike image) if you take the wrong turn—that should help you always recall a par-

Dendritic
Pertaining to a dendrite, that portion of a neuron that carries nerve impulses to the cell body; it is usually branched, like a tree.

ticular portion of the directions. Or picture how disappointed your significant other will be if you forget to bring home dinner—that should help you remember to get it.

- **Chunking information:** We chunk it, our brain doesn't chuck it! Break down memories into bite-sized pieces. For example, most people are only able to remember seven bits of memory, like a phone number, at any given time. So if you have to remember fourteen different names, learn them seven at a time. This is why making outlines or overviews *before* we dig into details helps us learn and remember better.

- **Concentration:** Concentration is the act of thinking, reading, or learning when our mind is totally, and actively, engaged. It takes willpower but is well worth it, when practiced regularly. According to Dr. Khalsa, "being able to achieve a high level of concentration is largely a result of having a healthy brain, full of physical energy."

- **Conscious forgetting:** Filter, filter, filter. It makes sense to consciously forget trivial details since they clutter the mind. Our senses do it as part of sensory discrimination; we should do it as part of what we might call cognitive discrimination. Working memory, the brain's version of RAM, always seems to be in short supply, so use systems to keep stock of small details. For example, write things down so that you can dispose of certain details until they are needed. Write down your schedule. Keep things in their correct places—your keys, your purse or wallet. Make lists, write notes, maintain files. Filter, filter, filter.

- **Many paths lead to Rome:** If all roads lead to Rome, certainly many paths lead to memory. The more associations we attach to each memory, such as a client's name, the more neural, or dendritic, pathways we will have to the memory of that client's name: her husband's name, her job title, the color of her car, or her hometown. This is a way of storing and remembering a memory via multiple channels—creating side doors to a memory that may stump us if we just try to remember her name and draw a blank.

- **Multiple encoding:** Encode your memory with more than just one sense. Say a phone number aloud, see it, and write it down. Three senses have now each encoded this phone number. This is why hands-on learning works so well with children, since their language centers are not yet fully developed. Smell is a very powerful way to encode memories, too—smells go directly to the hippocampus in the brain without having to go through the hypothalamus the way other sensory input does. So maybe spray some perfume on that phone number of your girlfriend after you write it down and look at it—just make sure that it's her perfume you're using!

- **PQRST:** A simple study method is known as PQRST: Preview, Question, Read, State, and Test. This method is a way to improve our recall of everything we read. Here's how we can use it:

  1. *Preview:* Before reading an article, quickly scan it, maybe picking up only the first and last paragraphs and the first line of every paragraph. Form a "preview" idea of what the article is about and what it's probably going to tell you.

  2. *Question:* Ask yourself, *What do I already know about this topic? Have I read about it before? What questions do I have about this subject that I hope this article answers?*

  3. *Read:* Actively read the article, keeping in mind the questions you hoped would be answered.

  4. *State:* After you have finished the article, review it, remembering what you already know about the subject and asking yourself if the article ultimately answered the questions you had in mind about the topic.

  5. *Test:* Quiz yourself on your memory of the article you just read.

- **Review:** Repetition, repetition, repetition. If you review something three times well, you will be not only three times more able to remember what you read but actually about twenty times better equipped to remember it, since repetition brings into play a memory function called long-term potentiation. Suffice it to say that those three separate reviews will anchor the memory better than one long, torturous "cram" reading.

The Mind-Body Connection and the Brain

Dr. Khalsa explains the mind-body/brain connection this way: "You are physically composed of electrons, protons and neutrons, all of which are moving constantly and consistently within your 30 trillion cells. Your body is, in effect, 30 trillion 'dancing cells of light' . . . thus, you possess a high degree of energy potential at the cellular level."

Many experts believe that mind-body exercises effectively shift, or rebalance, tremendous quantities of energy to the brain and endocrine systems, enabling the brain and body to use that energy better.

Mind-body exercises, such as the meditative yoga exercise known as the kirtan kriya, are designed to channel blood flow directly to the brain, making them, some argue, even better brain-circulation enhancers than cardiovascular exercise.

Depression and the Brain

Let's say you're exhausted from work. The body's symptoms of fatigue very much resemble depression, especially considering the brain's "trembling web" of overlapping connections that tend to activate each other. For instance, your down mood can be activated because your brain relates the body's symptoms of extreme fatigue with those of depression. This bottom-of-the-barrel mood in turn causes your thought processes to be clouded over. The fact that your thinking is not clear causes your mood to get even worse, and a vicious brain-drain and depression cycle emerges.

Psychological testing proves, as Dr. Victoroff

explains, that "depression hobbles memory." Brain scans using positron emission tomography show that depression slows brain metabolism.

As Victoroff writes, "The evidence that low mood is bad for the brain should drive a serious reassessment of our public health priorities. The value of mental health is not just a matter of life satisfaction; it may be a matter of the [brain's] survival."

Love and the Brain?

Dr. Robertson explains than when young rats are regularly stroked on the back with a soft, dry paintbrush, their adult brains develop better than do those of rats that as babies did not get this soothing stimulation. Research shows that "stroking alters the trembling web, and with these brain changes comes better brain functioning."

In studies of children who were institutionalized before age two versus children who were in a loving family from birth, test scores and emotional scores were much better in the never-institutionalized kids. However, the differences were no longer significant in those children who were adopted early by a loving family.

As Robertson added, "It is not only children's brains and bodies that thrive on love. It is just as true for adults, like you and me."

CHAPTER 8

PHYSICAL ACTIVITY AND DIET

Next to your muscles, the brain is the greatest consumer of sugar (glucose). It was once believed that the brain was a VIP organ—that it could get all of the glucose it needed regardless of what was happening in the rest of the body. In recent years, however, this concept has changed as our knowledge of the brain has increased.

For example, it is now known that the body's ability to get glucose from the blood to the tissues—including the brain—is impaired in diabetes and insulin resistance. Since the hippocampus, in the brain, is especially prone to glucose-deficiency damage, if glucose is not getting to this portion of the brain, then wasting away of this region may occur.

Insulin Resistance
A prediabetic condition in which insulin levels are elevated, but the insulin cannot efficiently transport blood sugar to cells.

According to a study published in February 2003 in the *Proceedings of the National Academy of Sciences*, NYU School of Medicine researchers led by Dr. Antonio Convit found that "an inability to quickly bring down high levels of sugar in the blood is associated with poor memory and may help explain some of the memory loss that occurs as we age."

"We have demonstrated that impaired glucose regulation is associated with memory [decline] and shrinkage of the hippocampus," says Convit.

"Our study suggests that this [glucose problem] may contribute to the memory [decline] that occurs as people age, and it raises the intriguing possibility that improving glucose [functioning] could reverse some of the age-associated problems [related to] cognition."

Your Brain and the Glycemic Index

Problems arise, however, when you eat too much sugar or foods with a high glycemic index (GI). The GI of a food is a measurement of how much and how fast your blood sugar rises in response to that food.

Researchers came up with an extensive list of foods that have a devastating impact on both blood glucose and insulin (where metabolism is happening), and published their results in the *American Journal of Clinical Nutrition* in 1997. They found, for example, that sugar and white bread have a GI of approximately 100. Rice, even brown rice, has a very high GI, too. Some foods you would never suspect, such as potatoes, cantaloupe, watermelon, honeydew, very ripe bananas, grapes, and all fruit juices have a high GI. Other fruits such as oranges, grapefruit, apples, berries, pears, peaches, and papayas have a moderate GI and are fine. All protein foods have a low GI; vegetables and salad are low, as well.

As far as carbohydrates go, yams, sweet potatoes, beans, and lentils are low while corn, pumpkin, beets, and other root vegetables are moderate and can all be included. Whole grains such as buckwheat (kasha), and bulgur wheat either as pasta or just cooked, are fine, as well. As a basic rule of thumb, keep away from "white" foods.

The problem with constantly eating high-GI foods, day in and day out, is that they significantly raise your risk for diabetes and insulin resistance (or Syndrome X). And they also make you gain weight. The type of weight gain associated with this sort of eating is the beer-belly look, when fat is deposited around the abdomen. This type of fat deposition is very dangerous and raises the risk of heart disease and stroke.

Sugar, Insulin, and Your Brain

So how does this way of eating adversely affect the brain? When you eat a high-GI food, your blood sugar goes up very quickly, and so does your insulin. Insulin's job is to escort glucose into working muscles and also to help facilitate the glucose into your brain. When both your insulin and blood sugar (glucose) rise very quickly, however, a metabolic switch is thrown that puts you into fat storage mode.

Also, the fast rise in insulin lowers blood sugar too quickly, because a large amount keeps getting pumped out by your pancreas; this in turn may cause hypoglycemia. Have you noticed after consuming lots of sugar, such as cake or cookies or a soda (nondiet), you "crash and burn" in about one hour? Have you experienced brain fog around 3 P.M.? This happens because your sugar drops due to what you ate at lunch. Skipping meals can cause the same brain fog and adversely affect your mental clarity, as well. You need to keep a constant fuel supply available to your brain for optimal performance.

One of the factors that lower the GI of a carbohydrate is fiber. Fiber can improve your handling of glucose, improve your insulin sensitivity, and stabilize your blood sugar. But the most important thing about these types of foods is that some of the complex carbohydrates in them acts like timed-release energy. Complex carbohydrates take some time to digest. So rather than raising your blood sugar quickly, the sugar is released from these foods at a much slower rate. They are the best way to keep a constant supply of glucose to your brain without the risk associated with high-GI foods.

This way of eating is the diet our ancestors followed. Unlike today, our ancestors could not buy prepackaged processed and junk foods, they did not eat cookies and cake, and they did not eat white bread or drink soda.

Pro-Brain Eating

Swiss researchers, in 2002, published the results of a study looking at healthy males, mental function, and types of diets. Their findings suggest, say the authors, that a protein-rich or balanced meal "seems to result in better overall cognitive performance, presumably because of less variation in glucose" processing.

Another study, this time in animals in 1996, found that a low-fat diet doesn't "do anything to preserve memory." Although not speculated upon by the authors at the time, we now know that diets rich in omega-3 fats (those found in fish and olive oil, for example) and low in cheap oils (such as soybean and tropical fats) and trans fats (such as those found in deep-fried foods and traditional tub margarine) reduce the burdens of "bad fat" breakdown products that are harmful and contribute to brain fog and mental decline.

Brain Health and Today's Disease Epidemics

The U.S. Centers for Disease Control and Prevention (CDC) estimates that seventeen million Americans have diabetes. Diagnosed in eleven million people and undiagnosed in approximately six million others, 8.6 percent of all Americans aged twenty through sixty-four have diabetes. In fact, diabetes is the sixth leading cause of death, and people with diabetes are twice as likely to die prematurely than are those without the disease.

The World Health Organization (WHO) estimates that the global diabetes figure could reach 300 million people by 2025. There is a growing recognition of the fact that there are 95 million Americans with some degree of insulin resistance, 102 million adults at risk for cardiovascular disease (CVD), and 108 million people who are overweight.

The United States is one of the fattest nations on Earth—and our children are not faring much better. In fact, over the last twenty-five years, the number of children who are overweight has tripled—22 percent of kids are overweight. Not only that, 13 percent of children aged six through eleven and 14 percent of kids aged twelve through nineteen are obese. And what is worse yet: 60 percent of overweight children aged five through ten have at least one risk factor for CVD; 25 percent have two or more risk factors. Tied to obesity, sugar-packed diets, and physical inactivity, type 2 diabetes—which used to develop almost exclusively in adulthood—is now the new children's epidemic.

The Bottom Line on Your Diet

We're not saying you can never cheat! What we are saying is that cleaning up your diet is an important factor in improving your brain function.

Exercise and the Brain

We know that you may not want to hear it, but exercise is critical as well. It improves the handling of blood sugar, decreases insulin resistance, and reduces the type of body weight that accumulates mainly as fat. Exercise also improves brain function.

Exercise is believed to improve memory and slow down memory loss in two ways. First, exercise improves overall health, which improves all mental functions, including memory; second, it combats stress and depression, both of which interfere with memory and contribute to cognitive decline.

The best place to start is to train aerobically. This includes any continuous movement such as brisk walking; using treadmills, indoor or outdoor bicycles, or stepper machines; low-impact aerobic workouts; and dancing. A good way to start is with five minutes every other day the first week; then add one to two minutes each week. The goal is to do the exercise continuously for at least thirty minutes, three times each week. Yes, five times each week is better!

Once you have become aerobically fit, it is important to do some strength training exercises. This can be done at home or in a gym with light weights, to start, or with exercise bands. If you haven't done any strength training before, we suggest either working with a trainer initially to make sure you are doing the movements properly or getting an exercise tape that incorporates strength training and teaches you how to use either bands or light weights properly. This type of exercise also improves the body's handling of blood sugar, decreases insulin resistance, and reduces body weight predominantly as fat. Even more important, muscle dictates your metabolism—so strength training can improve your ability to burn calories and body fat. It's also a good idea to let your family healthcare practitioner know about your planned exercise program.

Take Your Brain for a Walk

In a study by Dr. Kristine Yaffe that was presented at the American Academy of Neurology's Fifty-third Annual Meeting, May 5–11, 2001, in Philadelphia, Pennsylvania, the cognitive abilities of 5,925 women aged sixty-five and older were tested once, and then retested six to eight years later.

The results? Women who walked regularly were less likely to experience memory loss and mental decline associated with aging. Dr. Yaffe uncovered that, for every extra mile walked per week, "there was a 13 percent less chance of cognitive decline."

"You don't need to be running marathons," adds Dr. Yaffe. "The exciting thing is that there was a 'dose' relationship which showed that while even a little is good, more is better."

Physical activity was measured by the number of blocks walked per week and also by the number of calories used in walking, recreation, and stair climbing. The activity chosen really didn't matter, since the results were almost identical when Yaffe's team measured the total number of calories burned. Examples of moderate activities that reduced risk included playing tennis twice per week, walking a mile a day, or playing golf once per week.

You Can Do It!

With diet and exercise as a foundation, the brain-boosting supplements in this book can then be selectively incorporated into your brain- and health-optimizing program. The following chapter will help you do just that.

CHAPTER 9

CHOOSING THE RIGHT BRAIN-BOOSTING SUPPLEMENTS

Chapters 1 through 8 have offered you what we hope is a concise, practical little guide to memory-boosting supplements. But you don't have to go out now and buy *all* of the supplements listed in this book; in fact, we recommend against that approach. What we do recommend is that you start out with a premium-quality multivitamin and mineral supplement found at a health food store, preferably one that includes the ranges of antioxidant vitamins and B vitamins discussed in Chapters 2 and 3. Selectively begin with ginkgo-ginseng, and observe the improvements after several weeks. If you desire better results, try acetyl-L-carnitine, wait a few weeks, then try vinpocetine. Wait some more, then give alpha lipoic acid or huperzine A and some of the other supplements a shot.

Never take everything at once, or exceed the dosage ranges on the bottles. Otherwise you may find that you don't know which of what you're taking is helping you, or your liver will become overburdened with all these pills, or there will develop a mishmash of conflicting effects that cancel each other out. Another approach (which can be combined with the above) is to see which of the supplements discussed helps with a specific area that you are most concerned about, then give that supplement a try for several weeks first.

Nothing—no supplement, drug, or food—is a magic bullet. Please keep this in mind, so to speak. We have pored through literally hundreds of research papers and presentations filtered through the lens of what I (SL) know works from my active private nutritional practice and I (JG) know works from having talked to companies, health food retailers, and supplement consumers for more than eight years.

As far as which brands to buy, we recommend that you invest in purchasing supplements from the companies that have done the lion's share of the research.

For vitamins, we have emphasized in this book the importance of natural-source vitamin E. Carlson Laboratories is one company I (JG) have personally visited, and I can vouch for this firm's quality—although there are other fine manufacturers out there that you may also know and trust.

In terms of herbs, we mentioned Pharmaton and Nature's Way as excellent companies that have done a great deal of the research into herbs and herbal combinations. Wakunaga, Nature's Herbs, Enzymatic Therapy, Country Life, and Herb Pharm are other firms that produce herb-based supplements whose facilities we have visited and were impressed with.

As far as specialized supplements go, Pycnogenol (available through different distributors and manufacturers) appears to have the most research in the OPC area. Nevertheless, there are other types of OPCs, including ingredients derived from grapes, that science is beginning to support.

When choosing supplements, also look for any (or some) of the following seals. These are your guarantee that quality and purity standards were adhered to in terms of facilities, processing, manufacturing, and other factors:

- NNFA GMP (National Nutritional Foods Association's Good Manufacturing Practices)

- GMP (Good Manufacturing Practices)

- USP (United States Pharmacopeia)

- USP-NF (USP—National Formulary)

- ISO (International Standards Organization)

- NSF (National Sanitary Foundation)

If a manufacturer has adhered to one or more of these standards, then this will give you added assurance that you are purchasing a safe, quality supplement.

CONCLUSION

If you take nothing else from this book, please remember this: the *User's Guide to Brain-Boosting Supplements* that you hold in your hands right now is not about problems—it is about *solutions*. It is not about frustration, but about *success*. Not about losing it, but about *gaining* something, a very important something indeed—better memory and brain power that will enrich your life today, and for a lifetime.

It is our hope that this book has helped you learn about brain-boosting improvements—including diet, physical and mental exercises, and nutritional supplementation—that have a solid foundation in the science of nutrition. As we have outlined, modern nutritional science is uncovering the many nutrients and compounds that can selectively, and effectively, improve your mental powers, including antioxidants, herbs, and other targeted dietary supplements.

You have learned that the more you use your brain—consistently over time—the longer you will be able to hold on to it! As neurologist Jeff Victoroff says, we should seek out and embrace new things—or, as he puts it, "[dive] into new seas of neural natation." Active, deliberate learning appears to powerfully challenge the human brain, especially if it is enjoyable enough to regularly keep us motivated and engaged.

As we saw earlier, Dr. Victoroff invites us to

engage in a variety of pro-brain attitudes and activities, with this call to action paramount: Care passionately about what you learn and apply it *daily* in a "newly challenging lifestyle."

Today science suggests that a protein-rich, or balanced, meal results in better overall cognitive performance than does a low-fat or high-carb meal, presumably because there's less variation in glucose processing.

As we've also learned, physical exercise helps the old noggin, too—it improves the handling of blood sugar, decreases insulin resistance, and reduces body fat. "[You] don't need to be running marathons," says Dr. Kristine Yaffe. "The exciting thing is that there [is] a 'dose' relationship which showed that while even a little is good, more is better."

Optimizing your lifestyle—via diet, exercise, and supplementation—is absolutely critical, not only for a better-functioning brain, but also for your overall health and well-being. You'll feel great, you'll look great, and these types of changes represent the very best brain-focused antiaging "medicine" available.

SELECTED
REFERENCES

Aisen, PS, et al. A pilot study of vitamins to lower plasma homocysteine levels in Alzheimer disease. *American Journal of Geriatric Psychiatry*, 2003; 11(2):246–249.

Alive Books. *Encyclopedia of Natural Healing*. Second edition. Burnaby, BC, Canada: Alive Publishing Group, 1997.

American Academy of Neurology. Walking protects women from cognitive decline [press release]. May 8, 2001.

American Botanical Council. *Herbal Medicine—Expanded Commission E Monographs*. Austin, TX: American Botanical Council, 2000.

American Stroke Association. Ginseng may improve memory in stroke dementia patients: American Stroke Association meeting report [press release]. February 14, 2003.

Balch, PA, and Balch, JF. *Prescription for Nutritional Healing*. Third edition. New York: Avery-Penguin, 2000.

Birkmayer, GD, et al. [Stabilized NADH (ENADA) improves jet lag–induced cognitive performance deficit.] *Wiener medizinische Wochensshrift* [article and journal name in German], 2002; 152(17–18):450–454.

Cotman, CW, et al. Brain aging in the canine: a diet enriched in antioxidants reduces cognitive dysfunction. *Neurobiology of Aging*, 2002; 23(5):809–818.

Dimpfel, W, et al. Source density analysis of functional topographical EEG: monitoring of cognitive drug [DMAE] action. *European Journal of Medical Research*, 1996; 1(6):283–290.

Duke, JA. *Dr. Duke's Essential Herbs*. Emmaus, PA: Rodale Reach, 1999.

————. *The Green Pharmacy.* Emmaus, PA: Rodale Press, 1997.

Fairfield, KM, and Fletcher, RH. Vitamins for chronic disease prevention in adults: scientific review. *JAMA,* 2002; 287(23):3116–3126.

Fischer, K, et al. Carbohydrate to protein ratio in food and cognitive performance in the morning. *Physiology and Behavior,* 2002; 75(3):411–423.

Fukui, K, et al. Cognitive impairment of rats caused by oxidative stress and aging, and its prevention by vitamin E. *Annals of the New York Academy of Sciences,* 2002; 959:275–284.

Gormley, JJ. *DHA, A Good Fat—Essential for Life.* New York: Kensington Books, 1999.

Grodstein, F, Chen, J, and Willett, WC. High-dose antioxidant supplements and cognitive function in community-dwelling elderly women. *American Journal of Clinical Nutrition,* 2003; 77(4):975–984.

Healthnotes, Inc. *The Natural Pharmacy.* Second edition. Rocklin, CA: Prima Publishing, 1999.

Jelicic, M, et al. Effect of low levels of serum vitamin B_{12} and folic acid on cognitive performance in old age: a population-based study. *Developmental Neuropsychology,* 2001; 20(3):565–571.

Khalsa, DS. *Brain Longevity.* New York: Warner Books, 1997.

LeBars, PL, et al. Influence of the severity of cognitive impairment on the effect of the Ginkgo biloba extract EGb 761 in Alzheimer's disease. *Neuropsychobiology,* 2002; 45(1):19–26.

Lieberman, S, and Bruning, N. *The Real Vitamin & Mineral Book.* Third edition. New York: Avery-Penguin, 2003.

Lindemann, RD, et al. Serum vitamin B_{12}, C and folate concentrations in the New Mexico elder health survey: correlations with cognitive and affective functions. *Journal of the American College of Nutrition,* 2000; 19(1): 68–76.

Liu, J, et al. Delaying brain mitochondrial decay and aging with mitochondrial antioxidants and metabolites. *Annals of the New York Academy of Sciences,* 2002; 959:133–166.

Martin, A, et al. Effects of fruits and vegetables on levels of vitamins E and C in the brain and their association with cognitive performance. *Journal of Nutrition, Health & Aging*, 2002; 6(6):392–404.

Medical Economics. *PDR for Nutritional Supplements*. First edition. Montvale, NJ: Medical Economics Company, 2001.

MetLife Mature Market Institute. "Demographic Profile: The Baby Boomers in 2003." Undated, 2003.

Milgram, NW, et al. Landmark discrimination learning in the dog: effects of age, an antioxidant fortified food, and cognitive strategy. *Neuroscience and Behavioral Reviews*, 2002; 26(6):679–695.

Miller, AL. The methionine-homocysteine cycle and its effects on cognitive diseases. *Alternative Medicine Review*, 2003; 8(1):7–19.

Morris, MC, et al. Vitamin E and cognitive decline in older persons. *Archives of Neurology*, 2002; 59(7): 1125–1132.

Nilsson, K, et al. Improvement of cognitive functions after cobalamin/folate supplementation in elderly patients with dementia and elevated homocysteine. *International Journal of Geriatric Psychiatry*, 2001; 16(6): 609–614.

NYU Medical Center. High sugar levels linked to poor memory [press release]. February 3, 2003.

Paleologos, M, et al. Cohort study of vitamin C intake and cognitive impairment. *American Journal of Epidemiology*, 1998; 148(1):45–50.

Passwater, RA. *All About Pycnogenol*. Garden City Park, NY: Avery Publishing, 1998.

Reader's Digest Association. *The Healing Power of Vitamins, Minerals and Herbs*. Pleasantville, NY: The Reader's Digest Association, 1999.

Riviere, S, et al. Low plasma vitamin C in Alzheimer's patients despite an adequate diet. *International Journal of Geriatric Psychiatry*, 1998; 13(11):749–754.

Robertson, IH. *Mind Sculpture*. New York: Fromm International, 2000.

Rodale, JI. *The Complete Book of Vitamins*. Emmaus, PA: Rodale Books, 1970.

Rohdewald, P. A review of the French maritime pine bark extract (Pycnogenol), a herbal medication with a diverse clinical pharmacology. *International Journal of Clinical Pharmacology and Therapeutics,* 2002; 40(4):158–168.

Scholey, AB, and Kennedy, DO. Acute, dose-dependent cognitive effects of Ginkgo biloba, Panax ginseng and their combination in healthy young volunteers: differential interactions with cognitive demand. *Human Psychopharmacology,* 2002; 17(1):35–44.

Stipanuk, MH, ed. *Biochemical and Physiological Aspects of Human Nutrition.* Philadelphia: WB Saunders, 2000.

Veerendra Kumar, MH, and Gupta, YK. Effect of different extracts of Centella asiatica on cognition and markers of oxidative stress in rats. *Journal of Ethnopharmacology,* 2002; 79(2):253–260.

Victoroff, J. *Saving Your Brain.* New York: Bantam Books, 2002.

Virmani, MA, et al. The action of acetyl-L-carnitine on the neurotoxicity evoked by amyloid fragments and peroxide on primary rat cortical neurons. *Annals of the New York Academy of Sciences,* 2001; 939:162–178.

Wake Forest University. Wake Forest researchers ask: Can ginkgo prevent memory loss? [press release]. November 3, 1999.

Wang, LS, et al. Huperzine A attenuates cognitive deficits and brain injury in neonatal rats after hypoxia-ischemia. *Brain Research,* 2002; 949(1–2):162–170.

Wollschlaeger, B. Efficacy of vinpocetine in the management of cognitive impairment and memory loss. *Journal of the Nutraceutical Association,* 2001; 4(2): 25–30.

www.nutraingredients.com. A wise old herb [press release]. September 1, 2003.

Zhang, L, et al. Alpha lipoic acid protects rat cortical neurons against cell death induced by amyloid and hydrogen peroxide through the Akt signalling pathway. *Neuroscience Letters,* 2001; 312(3):125–128.

OTHER BOOKS AND RESOURCES

Barney, P. *Doctor's Guide to Natural Medicine.* Pleasant Grove, UT: Woodland Publishing Inc., 1998.

Challem, J, and Brown, L. *User's Guide to Vitamins and Minerals.* North Bergen, NJ: Basic Health Publications, 2002.

Challem, J, Berkson, B, and Smith, MD. *Syndrome X: The Complete Nutritional Program to Prevent and Reverse Insulin Resistance.* New York: John Wiley & Sons, 2000.

Glanz, K, Marcus Lewis, F, and Rimer B, eds. *Health Behavior and Health Education.* Second edition. San Francisco: Jossey-Bass, 1997.

Physical Magazine
Magazine oriented to body builders and other serious athletes.
Customer service:
1-800-676-4333
P.O. Box 74908
Los Angeles, CA 90004
Subscriptions: 12 issues per year, $19.95 in the U.S.; $31.95 outside the U.S.

The Nutrition Reporter™ newsletter
Monthly newsletter that summarizes recent medical research on vitamins, minerals, and herbs.
Customer service:
P.O. Box 30246
Tucson, AZ 85751-0246

e-mail: jack@thenutritionreporter.com

www.nutritionreporter.com

Subscriptions: 12 issues per year, $26 in the U.S.; $32 U.S. or $48 CNC for Canada; $38 for other countries.

INDEX

Printed in the USA
CPSIA information can be obtained
at www.ICGtesting.com
JSHW012007140824
68134JS00004B/49